BEDSORES:
Treatment, Prevention
& Home Remedies

About The Author

Harold David is a dermatologist, a consulting scholar and a social health advocate. His working experience traversed beyond several health institutions, research centers and colleges. He has lectured in several states in US on skin health care, natural healing techniques and clinical nutrition. In addition to his clinical work, he draws on his decades of experience as a yoga instructor, organic gardener, and spiritual seeker; he has lived in California and has traveled to many countries around the world.

CONTENTS

Bedsores

Bedsores are best regarded as ulcers that happen on areas of the body (skin) that are subjected to pressure which result from lying in bed, wearing a cast for a prolonged time or sitting in a wheelchair. Bedsores are also referred to as: **pressure injuries**, **decubitus ulcers**, **pressure sores** or **pressure ulcers**.

Bedsores' development are often common on skin that cover joints or bony areas of the body, such as the elbows, ankles, heels, tailbone, hips, shoulder blades, back of the head, or backs and sides of the knees. People that are likely at risk of bedsores have medical conditions that cause them to spend most of their time on a chair or bed, bedridden or otherwise not mobile, unconscious, or unable to feel and sense pain which can inhibit their ability to change positions. The risk increases if the person is not correctly positioned, turned, or provided with skin care and proper nutrition. People with circulation problems, high blood sugar level and malnutrition are at higher risk.

What Are The Likelihood of Developing Bedsores?

The likelihood of developing bedsores is greater if one has hindrance in movement in bed or changing of position while seated.

Other likely factors include:

- **Incontinence / Loss of Urine Excessively:** Tissues can become more liable to bedsores with higher exposure to urine and stool.
- **Immobility**: this simply refers to inhibition in movement. It might originate from poor health, spinal cord injury and others.
- **Health problems that can hinder blood circulation**: some of these health problems include; diabetes and heart (vessels like arteries and veins) related diseases, can increase the likelihood of tissue damage, which can in turn lead to bedsores.
- **Absence of Sensory Neurons for Perception:** neurological disorders and Spinal cord problems, can result to a loss of perception or

sensation. Ones inability to sense discomfort or pain can make one unaware of dangerous warning signs, possibly, if there is any need to change position on be or chair.

- **Malnutrition and hydration**: enough foods, fluids, proteins, calories, minerals and vitamins are needed in daily diets to sustain and maintain healthy tissues and to forestall any breakdown.

Bedsores Diagnoses and Stages

Doctors or health professionals diagnose bedsores by carrying out a thorough inspection of the skin of those that have symptoms related to them. They are classified into different stages in accordance with their physical appearance.

The doctor will likely examine your skin closely to ascertain if you have bedsores. If this is so, he'll assign a stage to the sore. Assigning a stage can help with the best treatment to administer. Blood tests might also be needed to carry out assessment overall health.

Some likely questions which your doctor/healthcare professionals might ask include:

- When did the bedsores first show up? Appearance? What's the level of the pain felt?
- Have you had bedsores in your past medical history? Can you relate the experience of how it was managed and treated? And what was the result of the treatment?
- Are you on any care assistance?

- What are your practices and procedures for changing of positions?
- Have you been diagnosed of any medical condition? What is your present treatment?
- What is your daily fluid intake diet?

Bedsores are classified into 4 different stages, from least serious to generally extreme or advance stage. These are:

- **Stage 1**: The skin area looks red colored and somehow feels warm when touched. In a person with darker skin, the area may have a purple or blue color. The individual may likewise complain of itches, burns and hurts.
- **Stage 2:** The skin area may have an open sore, scratch, rankle or blister. It looks 'damaged' in appearance. The individual whines of critical pain and the skin around the injury may lose color.

- **Stage 3**: The skin area has a crater-like display in appearance due to wounds beneath the surface of the skin.

- **Stage 4**: The skin area is seriously damaged, with the presence of a large wound. It can also involve bones, muscles, ligaments, joints and tendons. Bedsores infection is of critical risk at this stage.

Difficulty in full staging and evaluation of bedsore is very possible. Bedsores may be classified as "unstageable" when you have an eschar (which is a hard plaque with dark color) inside the sore. Sometimes your healthcare provider may request for surgical evaluation or further imaging to evaluate the full extent of the sore. The sore may also show *slough*, which is a discolored debris (tan, yellow, brown or green), which might make full evaluation more difficult.

Possible Complications of Bedsores

Bedsores, once formed on the skin can take maximum duration to heal. Infected bedsores can cause fever or chills; and take a time duration to heal and clear up. Uncontrolled spreads through the body lead to: generalized body weakness mental confusion and a rapid heartbeat rate.

Some other life-threatening complications associated with bedsores/pressure ulcers include:

- **Bone/Joint Infections**: An infection from bedsores can dig into the bones and joints. *Septic Arthritis,* a joint infection can damage tissue and cartilage. Also, a bone infection known as *Osteomyelitis* can limit the function of joints, arms or legs.

- **Cellulitis**: Cellulitis refers to a common infection of connected soft tissues the skin. Cellulitis can cause swelling and redness of the infected area, and can also cause warmth. People that suffer from nerve damage often do not feel pain in the skin area affected by cellulitis.

- **Cancer**: unhealed injuries and wounds can develop into a type of squamous cell carcinoma (characterized by scales).

- **Sepsis**: In rare occasions, bedsores can also lead to sepsis.

Simple Ways to Take Care of the Skin

The following suggestions are to be considered for skin care:

- **Maintain Clean and Dry Skin:** always use a gentle cleanser to wash the skin and pat dry. This cleansing routine should be carried out regularly to reduce the skin's vulnerability to urine, stool or moisture.

- **Protect the skin**: moisture barrier creams should be used for the skin protection from urine and stool. Change bedding if need be. Check for the wrinkles in the bedding or buttons on the clothing.

- **Carry out Daily Skin Inspection**: always take a close look at your skin daily for possible signs of a bedsores.

Best Ways to Prevent Bedsores

Bedsores can be prevented; also, existing sores can also be prevented from getting worse in the following ways:

- Carrying out routine inspection on the skin for areas of redness (a sign of breakdown of skin tissues) while paying rapt attention to bony areas like elbows, ankles, joints etc.

Other methods of preventing bedsores and preventing existing sores from getting worse include:

- Turning and changing position every 2 – 3 hours
- Sitting straight or upright on wheelchair, repositioning at most every 15 minutes
- Use soft padding on beds and wheelchairs. This reduces pressure.
- Always keep the skin clean and dry. Good skin care should be maintained.
- Eat good foods because bedsores can't heal without sufficient fluids, vitamins, proteins,

minerals and calories. Caring for the sores only without good nutrition won't heal the sores.

It is very possible to limit the risk of bedsores. When a sore is at an initial stage, one can treat it at home, but more advanced bedsores need professional care.

Home Remedies for Bedsores

(1)   **Turmeric:**   Turmeric   fast-track   the healing/recovery process of bed sores. It also possesses, anti-inflammatory and antiseptic properties that fight the infection and help the body deal with the sores or its symptoms.

> **Method 1:** use saltwater to clean the affected area. Then spray enough turmeric powder on the wound. Use clean bandage to cover the wound. This procedure should be repeated 3 times daily for quick healing.

> **Method 2:** you can also take warm turmeric milk 2 times in a day.

(2) **Aloe Vera:** aloe vera has high soothing and healing properties, it is useful in control of bedsore infection, keeps the infected skin moisturized, ensures speedy recovery and also aids healing.

Method 1: open the aloe vera leaf by cutting, then carry out extraction of the gel.

Method 2: Apply the gel extracted on the area of the skin affected, then, gently rub for a few minutes.

Method 3: leave for a while to dry on its own, then use a clean damp wool or cloth to wipe it off. Do this 3 times daily.

Method 4: You can also use aloe vera powder, cream, ointment or gel for healing.

(3) Honey: the natural antiseptic properties and can also work well on the skin with mild bed sores. It can reduce body itching, provide relief from injury, reduce risk of infection and helps in healing.

Method 1: Produce a thick mixture of honey and sugar in equal amounts. The mixture can now be applied on the affected body area, cover with a clean and soft bandage. Do this once in a day.

Method 2: pour honey on a very big banana leaf. Lie down, rest or sit back on this banana leaf for a number of hours. Do this daily.

(4) Coconut Oil: coconut oil have high abundance of medium-chain fatty acids, it improves blood circulation, keeps your skin in healthy state and also protect it from wound or damage that may result from bedsores.

Method 1: use warm coconut oil on all your limbs, back and legs.

Method 2: in a gentle way, massage well until the oil goes deep into the skin. **Method 3:** use 3 or 4 times in a day, prevent formation of new sores and to heal it.

(5) Comfrey Leafs: comfrey leaf is an herbal treatment for bedsores that is well known in alternative medicine. Comfrey leaves and roots are abundant in medicinal properties that can aid regeneration of tissues, reduction of inflammation or pain.

Method 1: Mix comfrey leaves (in powdered form) and slippery elm in equal ratio.

Method 2: Add some water to make into a paste.

Method 3: Use it on the sores, then cover it with a clean bandage.

Method 4: Let it stay overnight.

Method 5: The following morning, clean the wound with salt water. Do this every day.

(6) Saline Water: To aid bedsores healing, the surface should be cleaned with saline water (saltwater). Bedsores that are not properly cleaned are more susceptible to inflammation and infection. Saline water (saltwater) will lower excess fluid and also get rid of worn-out and damaged skin.

How are Bedsores Treated?

Healthcare professionals and care team provide specific treatment for bedsores depending on the stages and its severity.

Treating bedsores in early stages involve:

- Relieving or reducing pressure on the infected skin area. This is the first step, its strategies include:

  - Repositioning or by changing position: this is achieved by turning and changing your position often. How often you turn and change position is solely dependent on your condition and also the surface quality of the bed or seat you are on.
  - Usage of support surfaces: use bed, special cushions or mattress, this will help you lie or sit in a way that the vulnerable skin is best protected.

- Keeping the wound clean and taking proper care of the it

- Use special dressing or medicated gauze as protection. Special dressing that can be used for protection and to hasten up the healing process include:

  - Hydrocolloids dressings: it's made up of gel that aid the development of new skin cells in the sore, while keeping the healthy skin area dry.
  - Alginate dressings: they contain calcium and sodium. They're made from seaweed, and are known to hasten up healing process.
  - Others: like films, foams, antimicrobial/antibiotic, hydrofibres dressings can also be used.

You can always ask your care provider/physician about the dressing being used

- Infection prevention, pain control and,
- Maintaining good and healthy nutrition that contains sufficient protein and a good variety of

minerals and vitamins. This can speed up the healing process. Taking plenty of fluids is very significant, in order to avoid dehydration, because dehydration can slow down the recovery process.

Treatment of advance stages of bedsores (damaged skin) may be more difficult, it may involve any of the following methods:

- **Debridement:** which involves the removal of the damaged, dead or infected tissue. Small amount of dead tissue on the skin can be removed by using a specially designed dressings. Dead tissue in large amount can be removed by using: ultrasound, high-pressure water jets or surgical instruments such as forceps

- **Skin Grafts:** this involves transplanting/replacement of wound area with healthy skin. There are two common types of skin grafts: full-thickness and split-thickness and grafts.

A full-thickness graft involves replacement of the epidermis (which is the top layer of the skin) and dermis (which is the deeper layer of the skin) of the wound area. Healthy skin are usually taken from the forearm, collarbone, groin or abdomen. The skin taken are in smaller pieces, and the donor site are usually closed and joined together in a linear incision with staples or stitches. Full-thickness grafts are mostly used for small wounds on body parts that are visible, like the face. It blends well with the skin surface around them and always have an awesome cosmetic outcome.

On the other hand, split-thickness graft is typically used to cover wide wound areas. It also involves replacement of the epidermis and dermis of the wound area. This graft is said to be weak and has a smooth or shiny appearance. In split-thickness skin graft, healthy skin is usually taken from the abdomen, buttocks, outer thigh or back.

- **Surgery:** severe bedsore might not heal itself naturally. Surgery may be needed to close the wound, reduce the risk of infection and hasten up the healing process. Surgery process might be challenging, the risks associated with it might include:

  - Poisoning of blood
  - *Osteomyelitis,* an infection of the bone
  - Dying of implanted skin tissue
  - A painful collection of pus called *abscesses*
  - DVT known as Deep Vein Thrombosis, a blood clot in the brain

If surgery is recommended for you, ask the surgeon about the risks and benefits of the process.

- **Negative pressure wound therapy:** this is carried out by using an airtight covering on the wound and applying a vacuum to drain fluid

- **Medicine** (e.g. antibiotics to treat infections by stopping growth of bacteria)

- **Becaplermin Gel:** it is a new pharmacological active therapy which can help in treatment of diabetic skin ulcers.

Members of your care team might include:

- A physician who supervises the treatment plan

- A physician or nurse who specializes in wound treatment

- Medical assistants or nurses to provide both education and care for managing wounds

- A social worker who helps in addressing concerns related to emotions, long-term recovery or helps you access resources

- An occupational therapist (OT) who helps to provide rehabilitative care by ensuring suitable surfaces for seating or resting on

- A physical therapist (PT) who provide rehabilitative care, helps with improving body movement

- A dermatologist, a specialist doctor who manages and treats skin related conditions

- A dietitian who regulates and monitors your diets as well as nutritional needs

- An orthopedic surgeon, vascular surgeon, plastic surgeon or neurosurgeon

It's advisable to seek immediate medical attention if you show symptoms of infection, such as a fever, draining and smelling sores, increased redness of the wounds, swellings or warmth.

Doctors or other healthcare professionals always take close look at the sores before they'll will document its depth, size and how it respond to treatment.

Health Tips for You

Some tips that'll be of help when you visit your healthcare provider:

- Before you visit, jot down relevant questions you may have in mind
- Know the basis of your visitation
- Go with someone to help you ask related questions and take note of your provider's instructions.
- At the care center, jot down the name of any new medicines, treatments, diagnosis, and tests. Always write down new guidelines and instructions given to you by your provider.
- Inquire why a new treatment is recommended or medicine is prescribed, and also the side effects.
- Ask if there is possibility of treating your condition in other ways.
- Know reasons why a test is recommended and the interpretations of the results.

- Know the possible consequences of not taking the medicine or having the recommended test.
- In case you have a follow-up schedule, write down the purpose, date and time of appointments.
- Know the contact information of your healthcare provider, in case you have inquiry to make.